LECTIN FREE FOOD CHART

The Complete Guide With Low Lectin Food List And 14 Days Meal Plan To Lose Weight, Fight Inflammation And Improve Gut Health

ANGELA R. STATEN

TABLE OF CONTENTS

ABOUT THE AUTHOR

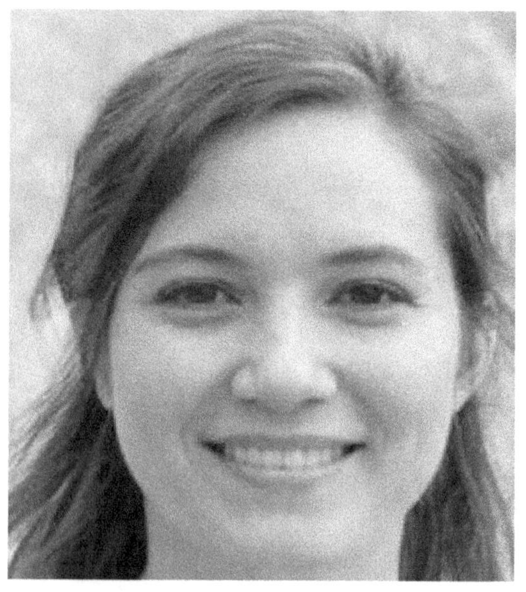

My name is Angela Rachel Staten, and I'm a medical professional and qualified nutritionist who is totally committed to using food as medicine.

Although it may sound generic, I have personally witnessed the profound impact that a healthy diet can have on people's lives.

I am a case study in action.

Whether you have lectin intolerance or are facing another health issue, my intention is not to give you a ton of confusing guidelines.

Rather, I wish to provide you with the means to effect long-term change.

One of the greatest methods to achieve this is by following a healthy diet, which focuses on eating tasty but simple foods that will fuel your body and provide you with the strongest defense against illness.

You will find in this book:

Clear explanations of the nutritional value of food and how it affects leading a healthy lifestyle.

scrumptious meals that genuinely inspire a desire for healthy eating.

Some pointers for incorporating this diet into your busy lifestyle.

Consider myself your companion in this. One delectable, nutritious meal at a time, I'm here to help you on your path to feeling better.

Let's get started.

INTRODUCTION

Have you ever been glued on a piece of toast that you could only imagine the uncomfortable afternoon that would surely follow?

Perhaps you have a strong desire for pasta, but the prospect of feeling bloated makes you grab for the salad.

You may be among the increasing number of people who are looking into lectin-free living if you are continuously navigating a maze of seemingly healthful meals that cause stomach problems.

Lectins are naturally occurring proteins that can be found in many plants and certain animals, despite the word itself sounding like something from a science fiction book.

Although lectins have a function in the world of plants, they can occasionally cause serious harm to our digestive systems.

The positive news is: You might finally be able to put an end to the frustration of having food allergies by learning about lectins and making dietary adjustments that will open up a world of delicious, gut-friendly meals.

This guide will help you understand the world of lectin-free foods. We'll go into the science of lectins, look at some unexpected foods that may contain them, and—most importantly—give you a useful manual for designing a tasty and sustainable lectin-free diet.

Prepare to be welcomed into a world of colorful, stomach-pleasing dishes and enjoy eating without worrying about discomfort!

What are lectins?

After eating something that seemed nutritious, have you ever had gas, bloating, or other digestive issues?

These uncomfortable feelings may be related to lectins, a class of proteins.

Lectins are naturally occurring, sugar-binding proteins found in a wide variety of plants, some animals, and even some fungi. In the plant world, lectins play a crucial role in defense – they act like tiny security guards, deterring insects and other herbivores from munching on them. Lectins bind to sugars on the surface of cells, which can have various effects depending on the type of lectin and the organism it encounters.

The intriguing element is that lectins have the ability to attach to carbohydrates in our digestive systems. Although most people's bodies can tolerate a certain amount of lectin exposure, some people may be more susceptible than others. This may result in a range of gastrointestinal discomforts, including:

- Swelling
- Gas
- Stomach ache
- Fatigue Diarrhea

It is significant to remember that lectins and their effects on human health are still being studied. Although some research points to a connection between lectins and digestive problems, additional research is required to completely grasp the cause-and-effect relationship.

So where in our diet are these "landmines" of lectin? Let's examine a few typical offenders in the upcoming chapter!

Why go lectin-free?

Recent years have seen a considerable increase in the popularity of the lectin-free diet, especially among those looking to reduce digestive issues and enhance general health. While studies are still being conducted, there are some possible advantages to using a lectin-free strategy that should be investigated. My responsibility as a health practitioner is to provide you with evidence-based knowledge so you may make well-informed dietary decisions.

Possible Advantages of a Diet Free of Lectin:

Enhanced Digestive Function: Research indicates that lectins may attach to the intestinal lining, which may cause inflammation and upset the digestive system. For people with sensitivity, cutting out lectin-containing foods may help with symptoms including gas, bloating, and abdominal pain.

Decreased Inflammation: According to several studies, lectins may be involved in the body's low-grade inflammation. A diet free of lectins has the ability to lower these inflammatory indicators, improving general health and lowering the chance of developing chronic illnesses.

Enhanced Nutrient Absorption: Some lectins have the ability to attach to important minerals, such as zinc, iron, and calcium, and obstruct their absorption. The body may be better able to utilize these essential nutrients if you follow a diet free of lectins.

Weight management: Whole, unprocessed meals are typically higher in fiber and more satisfying than processed foods. This is especially true of diets free of gluten. This may encourage the adoption of healthier eating habits and help with weight loss initiatives.

Crucial Points to Remember:

Tailored Approach: It's important to keep in mind that there may not be a single lectin-free diet that works for everyone. To ascertain whether this strategy fits with your unique requirements and health objectives, speaking with a registered dietitian can be helpful.

Adequacy of Nutrients: A carefully thought-out lectin-free diet can be high in nutrients, but it's crucial to be aware of any possible deficits. You can incorporate different sources of important vitamins and minerals with the help of your dietician.

Sustainability: A long-term sustainable diet plan is the most successful one. For some people, a balanced strategy that reduces lectins may be more maintainable than a rigid elimination diet.

Chapter 1

Learning About Lectin Content In Food

Many nutritious foods, like whole grains, legumes, and certain vegetables, contain lectins. These are naturally occurring proteins. While some research suggests lectins may have digestive effects in high amounts, they can also be beneficial. A well-balanced diet rich in these foods offers essential nutrients and shouldn't be completely avoided.

Cooking and Processing:

Fortunately, cooking methods like boiling and soaking can significantly reduce lectin levels in foods. So, a healthy diet that incorporates cooked legumes and whole grains is unlikely to contain concerning amounts of lectins.

Individual Needs:

If you suspect lectins are causing digestive issues, consulting a doctor or registered dietitian is crucial. They can help identify any potential food allergies, sensitivities, or intolerances. Restrictive diets like those eliminating all lectin-containing foods may not be suitable for everyone with digestive concerns. A personalized approach is key.

Foods to Avoid:

Category	Foods to Avoid
Grains	wheat, barley, rye, oats, corn, rice, quinoa, millet, sorghum
Legumes	beans, lentils, peanuts, soybeans, tofu, tempeh, edamame
Nightshade Vegetables	tomatoes, potatoes, white eggplant, peppers, goji berries
Most Fruits	(except berries: strawberries, blueberries, raspberries, etc.)
Dairy Products	cow's milk, yogurt, cheese, kefir (Goat and sheep dairy may be tolerated in some cases)
Seeds	cashews, sunflower seeds, pumpkin seeds, chia seeds
Sugary drinks and snacks	
Processed meats	

Foods to Include:

Category	Foods to Include
Protein	Pasture-raised meats (beef, chicken, lamb, pork), fish, seafood, eggs, bone broth
Fats	Avocado, avocado oil, coconut and coconut oil, olive oil, nuts (almonds, macadamia nuts, pecans), olives
Vegetables	Leafy greens (kale, spinach, collard greens), broccoli, Brussels sprouts, asparagus, celery, onions, mushrooms, artichokes, carrots, beets
Starches	Sweet potatoes, plantains, green bananas, turnips, parsnips
Fruits	Berries (strawberries, blueberries, raspberries, etc.)
Fats and Sweeteners	Limited amounts of healthy fats like avocado oil and olive oil. Sweeteners like stevia, erythritol, and monk fruit (in moderation)
Alternative Flours	Almond flour, coconut flour, tapioca flour, arrowroot flour

Remember:

This information is intended for general guidance and shouldn't replace personalized medical advice. See a medical expert if you have digestive issues. They can develop a plan that addresses your specific needs and ensures a balanced, nutritious diet.

Important Considerations:

Lectin content can vary within food groups. For example, some nightshade vegetables like bell peppers may be tolerated better than tomatoes or potatoes.

Cooking methods like soaking and boiling can reduce lectin content in some foods.

5 Simple Way To Reduce Lectin Content In Food

While some follow lectin-free diets, completely eliminating lectin-containing foods may not be necessary for everyone. The good news is, several cooking methods can significantly reduce lectin content in your favorite foods.

Here are some practical approaches:

1. Soaking:

This age-old technique is particularly effective for legumes like beans, lentils, and peas.
 Here's how to do it:

- ➢ Rinse your dry legumes thoroughly.
- ➢ Place them in a large bowl and cover them with at least three times their volume of water.
- ➢ Add a tablespoon of vinegar or lemon juice per cup of dry legumes (optional, may further enhance lectin reduction).
- ➢ Soak for a minimum of twelve hours, preferably overnight.
- ➢ Discard the soaking water and rinse the legumes again before cooking.

2. Sprouting:

- Sprouting grains, seeds, and legumes not only reduces lectins but also increases their nutritional value. Here's the basic process:
- Rinse your chosen grains, seeds, or legumes thoroughly.
- Place them in a jar or sprouting container with a mesh lid.
- Cover them with several times their volume of filtered water.

Soak for at least 8 hours.

- Drain and rinse the sprouts thoroughly two to three times a day.
- Continue rinsing and draining until sprouts reach your desired length (typically 1-3 days).
- You can then consume them raw, cooked in stir-fries, or added to salads.

3. Boiling:

- This simple method works well for some vegetables with moderate lectin content.
- Rinse your vegetables thoroughly.
- Heat up a big pot of water until it boils.
- Add the vegetables and cook them until tender-crisp.
- Drain the cooking water, as lectins leach out during boiling.

4. Pressure Cooking:

- Pressure cookers offer a time-saving alternative to soaking and boiling, especially for tougher vegetables and grains. They can also be more effective at reducing lectins.
- Follow your pressure cooker's instructions for cooking the desired food.
- Similar to boiling, discard the cooking water after pressure cooking.

5. Peeling and Deseeding:

- Lectins often concentrate in the peels and seeds of certain vegetables. Here's a simple tip:
- Peel vegetables like potatoes and cucumbers before cooking.
- Remove seeds from vegetables like peppers and squash before consuming.

Substitution For Common High Lectin Food

Following a lectin-free diet can restrict some common ingredients. However, there are delicious and nutritious alternatives you can explore! Here's a breakdown of substitutions for some high-lectin foods:

High Lectin Food	Lectin-Free Alternatives
Grains	
Wheat flour, barley, oats, rice	Almond flour, coconut flour, tapioca flour, arrowroot flour, cauliflower rice, spaghetti squash
Legumes	
Beans, lentils, peanuts, soybeans (tofu, tempeh)	Pasture-raised meats, fish, seafood, eggs, sprouted lentils (for better lectin reduction)
Nightshade Vegetables	
Tomatoes, potatoes, white eggplant, peppers	Leafy greens, broccoli, Brussels sprouts, asparagus, celery, onions, mushrooms, artichokes, carrots, beets, zucchini, yellow squash
Fruits	
All fruits except for berries	Berries (strawberries, blueberries, etc.), avocados
Dairy	
Cow's milk, yogurt, cheese	Unsweetened nut milks (almond, macadamia), unsweetened coconut milk, goat/sheep milk/yogurt (for some with tolerance)
Seeds	

Cashews, sunflower seeds, pumpkin seeds, chia seeds	Almonds, macadamia nuts, pecans, hemp seeds (limited amounts)
Sweeteners	
Refined sugar, honey (in large amounts)	Stevia, erythritol, monk fruit (use sparingly) pen_spark

Chapter 2

Lectin-Free Shopping List

Category	Items
Protein	Pasture-raised meats (beef, chicken, lamb, pork), fish and seafood (various types), eggs, bone broth
Fats	Avocado, avocado oil, coconut and coconut oil, olive oil, nuts (almonds, macadamia nuts, pecans), olives
Vegetables	Leafy greens (kale, spinach, collard greens), broccoli, Brussels sprouts, asparagus, celery, onions, mushrooms, artichokes, carrots, beets
Starches	Sweet potatoes, plantains, green bananas (for cooking), turnips, parsnips
Fruits	Berries (strawberries, blueberries, raspberries, etc.)
Fats and Sweeteners (limited amounts)	Avocado oil, olive oil, stevia, erythritol, monk fruit
Alternative Flours	Almond flour, coconut flour, tapioca flour, arrowroot flour
Seasoning	Iodized sea salt

Lectin-Free Pantry Staples

Category	Items
Protein Sources	**Fresh:** Pasture-raised meats, fish, seafood, eggs **Canned:** Wild-caught tuna, salmon (in water)
Healthy Fats	**Oils:** Avocado oil, olive oil, coconut oil **Nuts and Seeds:** Almonds, macadamia nuts, pecans, olives **Other:** Nut butters (almond, macadamia) – raw, sugar-free
Alternative Sweeteners (use sparingly)	Stevia powder, erythritol, monk fruit sweetener
Fats and Cooking Essentials	Bone broth, sea salt, black pepper, apple cider vinegar (optional), ghee or clarified butter (optional)
Starches (limited amounts)	Shirataki noodles, Green bananas (dried) for cooking
Alternative Flours	Almond flour, coconut flour, tapioca flour, arrowroot flour
Additional Considerations	Dried herbs and spices, frozen berries, unsweetened nut milks (optional)

Tips For Reading Food Labels And Identifying Lectin Content In Processed Foods

Lectin Sleuthing: How to Read Labels for a Lectin-Free Diet

Following a lectin-free diet requires vigilance when it comes to processed foods. While manufacturers aren't obligated to list lectin content, these practical tips can help you identify potential lectin offenders on food labels:

1. Focus on the Ingredient List:

This is your best bet for spotting lectin-containing ingredients.

Scan the list for hidden sources like:

Grains: Look for wheat, barley, oats, rye, corn (including corn flour, cornmeal, and cornstarch), and sometimes even rice flour (depending on processing).

Legumes: Be wary of ingredients like beans, lentils, peas, soybeans (including tofu, tempeh, and edamame), and peanuts.

Nightshade Vegetables: Watch out for tomatoes (including tomato paste, puree, and sauce), potatoes (including potato starch), white eggplant, peppers (all varieties), and sometimes even goji berries.

Other: Seeds (cashews, sunflower seeds, pumpkin seeds, chia seeds) might be listed as ingredients.

2. Ingredient Placement Matters:

Ingredients are listed in descending order by weight. So, if a lectin-containing ingredient appears near the beginning of the list, it's present in a higher quantity. This can help you prioritize products with lower lectin content.

3. Beware of "Sneaky" Names:

Manufacturers sometimes use unrecognizable terms for lectin-containing ingredients. Be familiar with aliases like "hydrolyzed vegetable protein" (often derived from soy) or "natural flavors" (which can sometimes include hidden lectins).

4. Check for Hidden Sugars:

While not directly related to lectins, added sugars can contribute to inflammation. Look for ingredients like "cane sugar," "high fructose corn syrup," and "brown rice syrup." Opt for products with minimal or no added sugar.

5. Consider Certifications:

Some brands offer products certified lectin-free. While not a foolproof method, it can be a helpful starting point, especially for pre-packaged snacks or condiments.

Remember:

Even "healthy-sounding" processed foods can contain hidden lectins. Reading labels diligently is crucial.

If you're unsure about an ingredient, don't hesitate to research it online or contact the manufacturer directly.

When in doubt, it's always better to err on the side of caution and choose a whole food alternative.

Chapter 3

A Guide to Stocking Your Lectin-Free Fridge

Following a lectin-free diet requires careful navigation when it comes to fruits, vegetables, protein sources, and storage methods.

This guide will equip you with the knowledge to make informed choices and maximize freshness.

Fruits and Vegetables:

Lectin-Free Choices:

Go Green: Leafy greens (kale, spinach, collard greens) are lectin-free superstars. Load up on these for essential vitamins and minerals.

Cruciferous Crunch: Broccoli, Brussels sprouts, cauliflower, and asparagus are all lectin-friendly and offer a variety of nutrients and fiber.

Rainbow Power: other colorful vegetables like carrots, beets, artichokes, and celery are lectin-free.

Sweet Treats: Berries (strawberries, blueberries, raspberries) are a delicious and healthy source of antioxidants.

Starchy Options: Sweet potatoes, plantains, green bananas (for cooking), turnips, and parsnips provide complex carbohydrates for sustained energy.

Minimizing Lectin Content:

Freezer Storage Tips:

Blanching for the Win: Blanch vegetables like broccoli, Brussels sprouts, and asparagus before freezing to preserve nutrients and extend shelf life (up to 12 months).

Berries on Ice: Flash-freeze berries on a baking sheet, then transfer them to airtight containers they can definitely stay for up to a year.

Frozen Chopped Herbs: Chop fresh herbs like parsley and cilantro, then freeze them in ice cube trays with olive oil for easy flavoring later (up to 6 months).

Protein Sources:

Lectin-Free Selections:

Meat: Pasture-raised options like beef, chicken, lamb, and pork are excellent protein sources with minimal lectins.

Fish and Seafood: A wide variety of fish and seafood like salmon, tuna, shrimp, and mussels offer healthy fats and protein, and are generally lectin-free.

Eggs: A complete protein source with minimal lectins.

Nuts and Seeds: Almonds, macadamia nuts, pecans, and hemp seeds are lectin-friendly options for healthy fats and protein.

Lectin Variations:

Beware of Cashews: While technically a nut, cashews are part of the legume family and contain higher lectin content. Avoid them on a strict lectin-free diet.

Limit Sunflower, Pumpkin, and Chia Seeds: These seeds contain moderate amounts of lectins. Consume them in moderation or avoid them entirely if strictly lectin-free.

Refrigerator Storage:

Fresh Meats: Store raw meat on the bottom shelf of your refrigerator to prevent drippings from contaminating other foods. Wrap them securely and use them within 3-5 days.

Fish and Seafood: Store fresh fish and seafood on a bed of ice in the coldest part of your refrigerator and consume within 1-2 days.

Eggs: Store eggs in their original carton on a shelf in the refrigerator, not the door, for up to 4 weeks.

Nuts and Seeds: Keep shelled nuts and seeds in airtight containers in the refrigerator for up to 3 months to prevent spoilage. Consider freezing them for longer storage (up to 1 year).

Remember:

Individual tolerances can vary. If you're unsure about a specific fruit, vegetable, or protein source, consult with a healthcare professional or registered dietitian.

Rotate your refrigerator and freezer stock regularly to ensure freshness and prevent waste.

Washing fruits and vegetables thoroughly before consumption is crucial for food safety.

Chapter 4

Lectin-Free Recipes for Every Meal

Category 1: Seafood Sensations

HERB-CRUSTED SALMON WITH ROASTED BRUSSELS SPROUTS AND AVOCADO SALSA

Yield: 2 servings | **Preparation Time**: 10 minutes | **Cooking Time**: 15-20 minutes

INGREDIENTS

- 2 salmon filets (about 6 oz each)
- 1/4 cup chopped fresh herbs (such as parsley, dill, and thyme)
- 1 tablespoon almond flour
- 1 tablespoon olive oil
- 1/2 teaspoon garlic powder
- 1/4 teaspoon paprika
- To taste, add black pepper and iodized sea salt.
- 1 pound Brussels sprouts, trimmed and halved
- 1 ripe avocado, pitted and diced
- 1/4 cup chopped red onion
- 1 tablespoon lime juice
- 1/4 cup chopped fresh cilantro

PREPARATION METHOD

1. Preheat the oven to 400°F (200°C). Put parchment paper on one side of a baking sheet.

2. In a small bowl, combine herbs, almond flour, olive oil, garlic powder, paprika, and sea salt.

3. Salmon should be patted dry before being placed on the baking pan. Spread the herb mixture evenly over the salmon filets.

4. Toss Brussels sprouts with a drizzle of olive oil and season with sea salt and pepper. On the baking sheet, distribute them across the salmon.

5. Bake for 15-20 minutes, or until the salmon is cooked through and the Brussels sprouts are tender-crisp.

6. While the salmon and Brussels sprouts are baking, prepare the avocado salsa. In a bowl, combine diced avocado, red onion, lime juice, and cilantro. Season with salt and pepper to taste.

7. Serve salmon and Brussels sprouts with a dollop of avocado salsa.

TIPS

- For a crispier salmon skin, preheat the oven to broil for the last minute or two of cooking.
- Feel free to substitute other fresh herbs for the ones listed.
- One tablespoon of dried herbs can be used in place of fresh herbs.
- To make the avocado salsa ahead of time, simply store it in the refrigerator with a squeeze of lime juice to prevent browning.
- **Lectin-Free Tip**: This recipe is naturally lectin-free as it avoids all high-lectin ingredients.

NUTRITIONAL INFORMATION

Calories: 450-500

Protein: 40-45 grams

Fat: 25-30 grams

Carbohydrates: 20-25 grams (including fiber)

Serving Size: 1 salmon filet with roasted Brussels sprouts and 1/4 cup avocado salsa

SPICY SHRIMP STIR-FRY WITH BROCCOLI AND COCONUT AMINOS

Yield: 4 servings | **Preparation Time:** 10 minutes | **Cooking Time:** 10-12 minutes

INGREDIENTS

- 1 pound shrimp, peeled and deveined
- 1 tablespoon arrowroot flour
- 1 tablespoon olive oil
- 1 pound broccoli florets
- 1 red onion, sliced
- 2 cloves garlic, minced
- 1 tablespoon grated ginger
- 1/2 cup coconut aminos
- 1/4 cup water
- 1 tablespoon sriracha (or to taste, omit for stricter lectin-free)
- 1 tablespoon lime juice
- 1/4 cup chopped fresh cilantro
- To taste, add black pepper and iodized sea salt.

PREPARATION METHOD

1. In a bowl, toss shrimp with arrowroot flour.
2. In a big wok or skillet, warm up the olive oil over a medium-high temperature.
3. Add shrimp and cook for 2-3 minutes per side, or until pink and opaque.
4. Take out and place the shrimp aside from the pan.
5. Add broccoli and red onion to the pan and cook for 3-4 minutes, or until broccoli is slightly tender-crisp.
6. Add garlic and ginger to the pan and cook for an additional minute, stirring constantly.
7. Stir in coconut aminos, water, sriracha (optional), and lime juice.
8. Simmer for approximately two minutes, or till the sauce begins to slightly thicken.
9. Put the shrimp back in the pan and toss to coat in sauce.

TIPS

- To make this dish even more lectin-free, omit the sriracha and use chopped red chili peppers instead (adjust the amount according to your spice preference).
- You can substitute other vegetables for the broccoli, such as asparagus, zucchini, or bell peppers (if tolerated).
- If you don't have arrowroot flour, you can use tapioca flour or almond flour as a substitute.
- Serve this stir-fry with a side of chopped avocado or mashed sweet potatoes for a more filling meal.
- Lectin-Free Tip: Coconut aminos are a good substitute for soy sauce in a lectin-free diet. Omit the sriracha for a stricter lectin-free approach.

NUTRITIONAL INFORMATION

Calories: 400-450

Protein: 40-45 grams

Fat: 20-25 grams

Carbohydrates: 20-25 grams (including fiber)

Serving Size: 1 serving with cauliflower rice (optional)

BAKED COD WITH LEMON AND ARTICHOKES

Yield: 2 servings | **Preparation Time:** 10 minutes | **Cooking Time:** 15-20 minutes

INGREDIENTS

- 2 cod filets (about 6 oz each)
- 1 tablespoon olive oil
- 1/2 teaspoon dried oregano
- 1/4 teaspoon garlic powder
- To taste, add black pepper and iodized sea salt.
- 1 lemon, thinly sliced
- One 14-oz can of drained and quartered artichoke hearts
- 2 spoon of sweet potato puree

PREPARATION METHOD

1. Preheat the oven to 400°F (200°C). Lightly grease a baking dish.
2. In a small bowl, combine olive oil, oregano, garlic powder, sea salt, and black pepper.
3. Pat cod filets dry and place them in the prepared baking dish. Use the olive oil mixture to lightly coat the cod filets.
4. Top the cod with lemon slices and artichoke hearts.
5. Bake for 15-20 minutes, or until the cod is cooked through and flaky.
6. During the last 5 minutes of baking, add the sweet potato puree,
7. Serve immediately.

TIPS

- You can use other white fish varieties, such as halibut or tilapia, instead of cod.
- For a richer flavor, add a tablespoon of chopped fresh thyme to the olive oil mixture.
- Serve this dish with a side of roasted vegetables or cauliflower rice for a complete meal.
- Lectin-Free Tip: This recipe is naturally lectin-free as it avoids all high-lectin ingredients.

NUTRITIONAL INFORMATION

Calories: 350-400

Protein: 40-45 grams

Fat: 20-25 grams

Carbohydrates: 15-20 grams (including fiber)

Serving Size: 1 cod filet with vegetables

THAI GREEN CURRY WITH SHRIMP AND BROCCOLI

Yield: 4 servings | **Preparation Time:** 10 minutes | **Cooking Time:** 15-20 minutes

INGREDIENTS

- 1 pound shrimp, peeled and deveined
- 1 tablespoon tapioca flour or arrowroot flour
- 1 tablespoon olive oil
- 1 pound broccoli florets
- 1 cup unsweetened coconut milk
- 2 tablespoons green curry paste (check label for lectin-free ingredients)
- 1 tablespoon fish sauce
- 1 tablespoon lime juice
- 1 tablespoon chopped fresh ginger
- 1 can (13.5 oz) coconut cream (full-fat, unsweetened)
- 1/4 cup chopped fresh basil (optional)
- To taste, add black pepper and iodized sea salt.

PREPARATION METHOD

1. In a bowl, toss shrimp with tapioca or arrowroot flour.
2. In a big wok or skillet, warm up the olive oil over medium-high temperatures.
3. Add shrimp and cook for 2-3 minutes per side, or until pink and opaque.
4. Take out and place the shrimp aside from the pan.
5. Add broccoli florets to the pan and cook for 3-4 minutes, or until slightly tender-crisp.
6. Stir in green curry paste, fish sauce, lime juice, and ginger. Stirring regularly, cook for a further minute.
7. Add coconut milk and coconut cream. After bringing to a simmer, cook for five minutes, or until the sauce starts to gradually thicken.

8. Return shrimp to the pan and heat through for 1-2 minutes.

9. Garnish with chopped fresh basil (optional) and serve over cauliflower rice (optional).

TIPS

- Choose a green curry paste that is lectin-free. Some brands may contain ingredients like tomatoes or legumes, so check the label carefully.
- You can adjust the amount of green curry paste depending on your desired spice level.
- For a richer flavor, add a tablespoon of chopped lemongrass to the pan with the ginger.
- Lectin-Free Tip: Ensure your green curry paste is lectin-free homemade and safe compared to store bought.

NUTRITIONAL INFORMATION

Calories: 150 (approx.)

Calories: 450-500

Protein: 40-45 grams

Fat: 25-30 grams

Carbohydrates: 20-25 grams (including fiber)

Serving Size: 1 serving with cauliflower rice (optional)

SHRIMP SCAMPI WITH SHIRATAKI NOODLES AND GARLIC

Yield: 2 servings | **Preparation Time:** 10 minutes | **Cooking Time:** 10-12 minutes

INGREDIENTS

- 1 pound shrimp, peeled and deveined
- 1 tablespoon olive oil
- 2 cloves garlic, minced
- 1/4 cup chopped fresh parsley
- 1/4 cup chopped fresh basil
- 1 tablespoon lemon juice
- To taste, add black pepper and iodized sea salt.
- 2 packages (7 oz each) shirataki noodles, drained and rinsed

PREPARATION METHOD

1. In a big skillet set over a medium-high temperature, warm up the olive oil.
2. Add shrimp and cook for 2-3 minutes per side, or until pink and opaque.
3. Take out and place the shrimp aside from the pan.
4. Cook the garlic in the pan for about thirty seconds or until it smells fragrant.
5. Stir in parsley, basil, and lemon juice. Cook for an additional minute.
6. Add shirataki noodles to the pan and toss to coat with the sauce. Heat through for 1-2 minutes.
7. Return shrimp to the pan and heat through for another minute.
8. To taste, add black pepper and sea salt for seasoning.
9. Serve immediately.

- You can add a splash of dry white wine to the pan with the garlic for extra flavor.

- If you don't have fresh herbs, you can use 1 teaspoon of dried parsley and 1/2 teaspoon of dried basil.

- For a creamier sauce, add a tablespoon of unsweetened coconut milk to the pan with the lemon juice.

- Lectin-Free Tip: This recipe is naturally lectin-free by omitting tomatoes, peppers, and other high-lectin ingredients.

NUTRITIONAL INFORMATION

Calories: 350-400

Protein: 40-45 grams

Fat: 15-20 grams

Carbohydrates: 10-15 grams (including fiber)

Serving Size: 1 serving

COCONUT CURRY MUSSELS WITH SWEET POTATO NOODLES

Yield: 4 servings | **Preparation Time:** 15 minutes | **Cooking Time:** 20-25 minutes

INGREDIENTS

- 2 pounds mussels, scrubbed and debearded
- 1 tablespoon olive oil
- 1 onion, chopped
- 2 cloves garlic, minced
- 1 tablespoon grated ginger
- 1 tablespoon green curry paste (check label for lectin-free ingredients)
- 1 can (13.5 oz) coconut milk (unsweetened)
- 2 cups cooked sweet potato noodles
- 1 cup chicken broth (or vegetable broth for a vegan option)
- 1 tablespoon fish sauce (optional)
- 1 tablespoon lime juice
- 1/4 cup chopped fresh cilantro
- To taste, add black pepper and iodized sea salt.

PREPARATION METHOD

1. In a big pot or Dutch oven, warm up the olive oil over a medium-high temperature.
2. Add onion and cook for 3-4 minutes, or until softened.
3. Stir in garlic and ginger and cook for an additional minute, or until fragrant.
4. Add green curry paste and cook for another minute, stirring constantly.
5. Pour in coconut milk and chicken broth. Bring to a simmer.
6. Add mussels, fish sauce (optional), and lime juice. Cover the pot and cook for 5-7 minutes, or until the mussels open. Discard any unopened mussels.
7. Stir in chopped cilantro and season with sea salt and black pepper to taste.
8. Serve immediately over cooked sweet potato noodles.

- For a smoother salsa, mash some of the avocado with a fork before combining with other ingredients.
- If the salsa isn't spicy enough, add a few extra sprinkles of chopped jalapeño.
- Serve immediately with plantain chips or your favorite lectin-free crackers.

NUTRITIONAL INFORMATION

Calories: 400-450

Protein: 40-45 grams

Fat: 20-25 grams

Carbohydrates: 30-35 grams (including fiber)

Serving Size: 1 serving with sweet potato noodles

SEARED CHICKEN WITH GARLIC GREEN BEANS AND MASHED SWEET POTATOES

Yield: 2 servings | **Preparation Time:** 10 minutes | **Cooking Time**: 25-30 minutes

INGREDIENTS

- 2 boneless, skinless chicken breasts (about 6 oz each), grass-fed (or pasture-raised)
- 1 tablespoon olive oil
- 1/2 teaspoon dried thyme
- 1/4 teaspoon garlic powder
- To taste, add black pepper and iodized sea salt.
- 1 pound fresh green beans, trimmed
- 2 cloves garlic, minced
- 2 large sweet potatoes, peeled and cubed
- 1/4 cup unsweetened nut milk (almond or macadamia)
- 1 tablespoon butter (optional)
- Chopped fresh chives (optional, for garnish)

PREPARATION METHOD

1. Pat chicken breasts dry and season generously with thyme, garlic powder, sea salt, and black pepper.
2. Pour the olive oil into a large skillet and heat it over medium-high temperature.
3. Add chicken breasts and cook for 5-7 minutes per side, or until cooked through.
4. Take out and set aside the chicken from the pan.
5. Boil some salted water in a pot whilst the chicken is cooking.
6. Add green beans and cook for 3-4 minutes, or until tender-crisp.
7. To end cooking, drain and rinse over cold water.
8. In the same pot used for green beans, add sweet potato cubes and enough water to cover. After bringing to a boil, lower the heat, and cook the sweet potatoes until they are soft, approximately fifteen to twenty minutes.
9. Drain the water.
10. Mash the sweet potatoes with nut milk and butter (optional) until smooth and creamy.

11. To taste, add more sea salt and pepper for seasoning.

12. Slice the cooked chicken breasts.

13. Serve chicken with mashed sweet potatoes and garlic green beans. Garnish with chopped fresh chives (optional).

TIPS

- You can use boneless, skinless chicken thighs instead of breasts.
- For extra flavor, marinate the chicken in your favorite lectin-free marinade for at least 30 minutes before cooking.
- Feel free to add other lectin-friendly vegetables to the green beans, such as asparagus, broccoli, or zucchini.
- Lectin-Free Tip: This recipe is naturally lectin-free by avoiding all high-lectin ingredients.

NUTRITIONAL INFORMATION

Calories: 500-550

Protein: 50-55 grams

Fat: 25-30 grams

Carbohydrates: 30-35 grams (including fiber)

Serving Size: 1 chicken breast with mashed sweet potatoes and green beans

COCONUT CURRY CHICKEN WITH CAULIFLOWER RICE

Yield: 4 servings | **Preparation Time:** 15 minutes | Cooking Time: 20-25 minutes

INGREDIENTS

- 2 boneless, skinless chicken breasts (about 6 oz each), grass-fed (or pasture-raised)
- 1 tablespoon olive oil
- 1 onion, chopped
- 2 cloves garlic, minced
- 1 tablespoon grated ginger
- 1 tablespoon green curry paste (check label for lectin-free ingredients)
- 1 can (13.5 oz) coconut milk (unsweetened)
- 1 cup chicken broth
- 1 tablespoon fish sauce (optional)
- 1 tablespoon lime juice
- 1/4 cup chopped fresh cilantro
- To taste, add black pepper and iodized sea salt.
- 1 head cauliflower, riced (or use pre-riced cauliflower)

NUTRITIONAL INFORMATION

1. Cut chicken breasts into bite-sized pieces.
2. In a big skillet or Dutch oven, warm the olive oil over a medium-high temperature.
3. Add onion and cook for 3-4 minutes, or until softened.
4. Stir in garlic and ginger and cook for an additional minute, or until fragrant.
5. Add green curry paste and cook for another minute, stirring constantly.
6. Pour in coconut milk and chicken broth. Bring to a simmer.
7. Add chicken pieces, fish sauce (optional), and lime juice. When the chicken is thoroughly cooked, simmer it in the covered pot for between fifteen and twenty minutes..
8. Stir in chopped cilantro and season with sea salt and black pepper to taste.
9. Serve chicken curry over cauliflower rice.

TIPS

- Choose a green curry paste that is lectin-free. Some brands may contain ingredients like tomatoes or legumes, so check the label carefully.
- You can adjust the amount of green curry paste depending on your desired spice level.
- For a thicker curry, simmer for a few minutes longer after adding the chicken.
- Lectin-Free Tip: This recipe avoids common lectin-containing ingredients like tomatoes and peppers. Ensure your green curry paste is lectin-free.

NUTRITIONAL INFORMATION

Calories: 450-500

Protein: 45-50 grams

Fat: 20-25 grams

Carbohydrates: 25-30 grams (including fiber)

Serving Size: 1 serving with cauliflower rice

TURMERIC-ROASTED CHICKEN WITH PARSNIPS AND CARROTS

Yield: 2 servings

INGREDIENTS

- 2 whole bone-in, skin-on chicken breasts (or 4 bone-in, skin-on chicken thighs)
- 1 tablespoon olive oil
- 1 tablespoon ground turmeric
- 1 teaspoon paprika
- 1/2 teaspoon garlic powder
- To taste, add black pepper and iodized sea salt.
- Two large parsnips, chopped into bits after peeling
- 2 large carrots, peeled and cut into chunks
- 1/4 cup of finely chopped parsley, if desired, for topping

PREPARATION METHODS

1. Preheat the oven to 400°F (200°C). Put parchment paper on one baking sheet.
2. In a small bowl, combine olive oil, turmeric, paprika, garlic powder, sea salt, and black pepper. Apply the spice mixture evenly over the chicken thighs or breasts.
3. Arrange the chicken on the prepared baking sheet. Scatter the parsnip and carrot chunks around the chicken.
4. Roast for 45-50 minutes, or until the chicken is cooked through and the vegetables are tender-crisp. The juices should run clear when the thickest part of the chicken is pierced with a knife.

5. Serve with a garnish of finely chopped fresh parsley, if desired.

TIPS

- You can add other lectin-friendly root vegetables to the roasting pan, such as turnips or sweet potatoes.
- For extra flavor, stuff the chicken cavity with chopped lemons or oranges before roasting.
- Lectin-Free Tip: This recipe is naturally lectin-free by omitting all high-lectin ingredients

NUTRITIONAL INFORMATION

Calories: 550-600

Protein: 60-65 grams

Fat: 30-35 grams

Carbohydrates: 30-35 grams (including fiber)

Serving Size: 1 chicken piece with roasted vegetables

SPICY CHICKEN LETTUCE WRAPS WITH SWEET POTATO FRIES

Yield: 2 servings | **Preparation Time:** 20 minutes | **Cooking Time:** 30-35 minutes

INGREDIENTS

For the Chicken:

- 1 pound boneless, skinless chicken breasts (about 2 breasts), grass-fed (or pasture-raised)
- 1 tablespoon olive oil
- 1 tablespoon coconut aminos (substitute for soy sauce)
- 1 tablespoon rice vinegar
- 1/2 teaspoon ground ginger
- 1 clove garlic, minced
- 1/2 teaspoon ground cumin
- 1/4 teaspoon paprika
- To taste, add black pepper and iodized sea salt.

For the Lettuce Wraps:

- One head of washed and separated romaine lettuce
- 1 avocado, diced
- 1/4 cup chopped red onion (optional)
- 1/4 cup chopped fresh cilantro
- Lime wedges (optional)
- For the Sweet Potato Fries:
- One large sweet potato, sliced into wedges after peeling
- 1 tablespoon olive oil
- 1/2 teaspoon ground cinnamon (optional)
- To taste, add black pepper and iodized sea salt.

PREPARATION METHODS

1. Marinate the Chicken: In a bowl, combine olive oil, coconut aminos, rice vinegar, ginger, garlic, cumin, paprika, sea salt, and black pepper. Toss to coat the chicken breasts after adding them. Marinate for at least 30 minutes, or up to overnight.

2. Prepare the Sweet Potato Fries: Preheat the oven to 400°F (200°C). Put parchment paper on one baking sheet. Toss sweet potato wedges with olive oil, cinnamon (optional), sea salt, and pepper. Spread them on the prepared baking sheet and bake for 20-25 minutes, or until tender-crisp, flipping halfway through.

3. Prepare the chicken: A big skillet or grill pan should be heated to medium to high temperature.

4. Remove the chicken from the marinade and cook for 5-7 minutes per side, or until cooked through. Slice the chicken after letting it rest for a few minutes.

5. Assemble the Lettuce Wraps: Arrange romaine lettuce leaves on a plate. Top with sliced chicken, diced avocado, red onion (optional), and cilantro. Drizzle with lime juice (optional) and serve with sweet potato fries.

TIPS

- You can use ground chicken or chicken thighs instead of breasts. Adjust cooking time accordingly.

- For a vegetarian option, substitute tofu or tempeh for the chicken and marinate it in the same way.

- Feel free to add other lectin-free vegetables to the lettuce wraps, such as shredded cabbage or chopped cucumber.

- Lectin-Free Tip: Substitute soy sauce with coconut aminos for the marinade. Omit sriracha for a stricter lectin-free approach.

NUTRITIONAL INFORMATION

Calories: 500-550

Protein: 50-55 grams

Fat: 25-30 grams

Carbohydrates: 30-35 grams (including fiber)

Serving Size: 2-3 lettuce wraps with sweet potato fries

ONE-PAN CHICKEN FAJITAS WITH ONIONS

Yield: 2 servings | **Preparation Time**: 10 minutes | **Cooking Time**: 20-25 minutes

INGREDIENTS

- 1 pound boneless, skinless chicken breasts (about 2 breasts), grass-fed (or pasture-raised)
- 1 tablespoon olive oil
- 1 tablespoon ground cumin
- 1 teaspoon chili powder
- 1/2 teaspoon smoked paprika
- 1/4 teaspoon garlic powder
- To taste, add black pepper and iodized sea salt.
- 1 large red onion, sliced
- 1/4 cup chopped fresh cilantro (optional, for garnish)

For Serving:

- Large flour tortillas (substitute with lettuce wraps or large romaine lettuce leaves for a lectin-free option)
- Guacamole (optional)
- Salsa (optional)
- Sour cream (optional - dairy may not be tolerated on a lectin-free diet)

PREPARATION METHODS

1. Preheat the oven to 400°F (200°C). Line a baking sheet with parchment paper.
2. In a bowl, combine olive oil, cumin, chili powder, paprika, garlic powder, sea salt, and black pepper. Add chicken breasts and toss to coat.
3. Arrange the chicken and sliced onion on the prepared baking sheet.
4. Roast for 20-25 minutes, or until the chicken is cooked through and the onions are tender-crisp.
5. Once cooked, slice the chicken into strips.
6. For Serving: Warm tortillas (optional - lectin-free option: use lettuce wraps or large romaine lettuce leaves), guacamole (optional), salsa (optional), and sour cream (optional - dairy may not be tolerated on a lectin-free diet).

7. Serve the chicken fajita mixture with your chosen toppings. Garnish with chopped fresh cilantro (optional).

TIPS

- You can use chicken thighs instead of breasts. Adjust cooking time accordingly.
- For extra flavor, marinate the chicken in the spice mixture for at least 30 minutes before roasting.
- Feel free to add other lectin-free vegetables to the baking sheet, such as chopped zucchini or yellow squash.
- Lectin-Free Tip: This recipe is easily adapted for a lectin-free diet by omitting peppers and using lettuce wraps instead of tortillas. Avoid using dairy products like sour cream unless tolerated in your specific lectin-free approach.

NUTRITIONAL INFORMATION

Calories: 400-450 (without tortillas or sour cream)

Protein: 45-50 grams

Fat: 20-25 grams

Carbohydrates: 15-20 grams (including fiber) (without tortillas)

Serving Size: 1 serving with chicken fajita mixture and chosen toppings (without tortillas or sour cream)

MARINATED CHICKEN FAJITA SALAD WITH CILANTRO LIME DRESSING

Yield: 2 servings | **Preparation Time:** 15 minutes | **Cooking Time:** 20-25 minutes

INGREDIENTS

For the Chicken:

- 1 pound boneless, skinless chicken breasts (about 2 breasts), grass-fed (or pasture-raised)
- 1 tablespoon olive oil
- 1 tablespoon lime juice
- 1 tablespoon ground cumin
- 1 teaspoon chili powder
- 1/2 teaspoon smoked paprika
- 1/4 teaspoon garlic powder
- To taste, add black pepper and iodized sea salt.

For the Salad:

- 2 cups mixed greens (such as romaine, arugula, spinach)
- 1 avocado, sliced
- 1/2 red onion, thinly sliced (optional)
- 1 cup chopped cucumber
- 1/4 cup crumbled feta cheese (optional - dairy may not be tolerated on a lectin-free diet)
- For the Cilantro Lime Dressing:
- 1/4 cup olive oil
- 2 tablespoons fresh lime juice
- 1 tablespoon chopped fresh cilantro
- 1 teaspoon honey (or substitute with another lectin-free sweetener like allulose)
- 1/2 teaspoon garlic powder
- To taste, add black pepper and iodized sea salt.

PREPARATION METHODS

1. Marinate the Chicken: In a bowl, combine olive oil, lime juice, cumin, chili powder, paprika, garlic powder, sea salt, and black pepper. Add chicken breasts and toss to coat. Marinate for at least 30 minutes, or up to overnight.

2. Prepare the chicken: A big skillet or grill pan should be heated to medium to high temperature. Remove the chicken from the marinade and cook for 5-7 minutes per side, or until cooked through. Slice the chicken after letting it rest for a few minutes.

3. Prepare the Salad: In a large bowl, combine mixed greens, avocado slices, red onion (optional), and cucumber.

4. Make the Cilantro Lime Dressing: In a small jar or bowl, whisk together olive oil, lime juice, cilantro, honey (or substitute), garlic powder, sea salt, and pepper.

5. Assemble the Salad: Top the salad greens with sliced chicken, crumbled feta cheese (optional), and drizzle with the cilantro lime dressing.

TIPS

- You can use chicken thighs instead of breasts. Adjust cooking time accordingly.
- For a vegetarian option, omit the chicken and add another lectin-free protein source like grilled tofu or tempeh.
- Experiment with other lectin-free vegetables in the salad, such as chopped bell peppers (if tolerated in your lectin-free approach), shredded carrots, or cherry tomatoes.
- Lectin-Free Tip: Substitute honey with another lectin-free sweetener like allulose in the cilantro lime dressing. Avoid using dairy products like feta cheese unless tolerated in your specific lectin-free plan.

NUTRITIONAL INFORMATION

Calories: 450-500 (without feta cheese)

Protein: 40-45 grams

Fat: 20-25 grams

Carbohydrates: 20-25

COCONUT FLOUR PANCAKES WITH MIXED BERRY COMPOTE

Yield: 2-3 servings | **Preparation Time**: 10 minutes | **Cooking Time:** 10-15 minutes

INGREDIENTS

For the Pancakes:

- 1 cup almond flour
- 1/4 cup unsweetened shredded coconut (optional)
- 1/4 teaspoon baking powder
- 1/4 teaspoon baking soda
- Iodized sea salt
- 3 large eggs
- 1/4 cup milk alternative (coconut milk, almond milk)
- 1 tablespoon melted coconut oil
- 1 teaspoon vanilla extract (optional)

For the Mixed Berry Compote (optional):

- 1 cup mixed berries (strawberries, blueberries, raspberries)
- 1-2 tablespoons water
- 1 tablespoon lemon juice (optional)
- Pinch of allulose or another lectin-free sweetener (optional)

PREPARATION METHODS

1. Prepare the Pancakes: In a bowl, whisk together almond flour, shredded coconut (optional), baking powder, baking soda, and sea salt.
2. In a separate bowl, whisk together eggs, milk alternative, melted coconut oil, and vanilla extract (optional).
3. Combine the wet and dry ingredients, mixing until just combined. Don't overmix.
4. Heat a lightly greased skillet over medium heat. Pour 1/4 cup batter per pancake.
5. Cook for approximately two to three minutes on each side, or until well cooked and golden brown.
6. When bubbles start to form on the surface, then flip.

7. For the Mixed Berry Compote (optional): In a small saucepan, combine berries, water, lemon juice (optional), and sweetener (optional). Heat over medium heat until the berries soften and release their juices, about 5 minutes. Mash slightly with a fork if desired.

TIPS

- For thicker pancakes, use slightly less milk alternative.
- Add a pinch of cinnamon or nutmeg to the batter for extra flavor.
- Top the pancakes with your favorite lectin-free toppings like sliced banana, additional berries, or chopped nuts (almonds, walnuts).
- Lectin-Free Tip: This recipe is naturally lectin-free by avoiding wheat flour and dairy. Substitute regular milk with a lectin-free milk alternative.

NUTRITIONAL INFORMATION

Calories: 300-350

Protein: 20-25 grams

Fat: 20-25 grams

Carbohydrates: 10-15 grams (including fiber)

Serving Size: 2-3 pancakes

FRITTATA WITH SAUTEED MUSHROOMS AND SPINACH

Yield: 4-6 servings | **Preparation Time:** 10 minutes | **Cooking Time:** 25-30 minutes

INGREDIENTS

- 8 large eggs
- 1/4 cup chopped fresh parsley
- To taste, add iodized sea salt and black pepper.
- 1 tablespoon olive oil
- 8 ounces sliced mushrooms (cremini, portobello, or your choice)
- 4 cups chopped fresh spinach

PREPARATION METHODS

1. Preheat the oven to 375°F (190°C). Grease a pie dish or skillet that is 10 inches and safe to use in the oven.
2. In a large bowl, whisk together eggs, parsley, sea salt, and black pepper.
3. Heat olive oil in the skillet over medium heat. Add mushrooms and cook until softened and golden brown, about 5 minutes.
4. Stir in the spinach and cook until wilted, about 2 minutes.
5. Over the sautéed veggies in the skillet, pour the egg mixture.
6. Bake for 20-25 minutes, or until the eggs are set and the center is no longer runny.
7. Let cool slightly before slicing and serving.

- For a vegetarian option, add crumbled cooked tempeh or chopped roasted vegetables to the egg mixture.
- Feel free to add other lectin-free vegetables to the frittata, such as chopped zucchini, diced bell peppers (if tolerated in your lectin-free approach), or chopped asparagus.
- Experiment with different herbs and spices in the egg mixture, such as chopped chives, dried thyme, or a pinch of nutmeg.
- Lectin-Free Tip: This recipe avoids tomatoes (typically used in omelets) and dairy (cheese).

NUTRITIONAL FACTS

Calories: 250-300

Protein: 20-25 grams

Fat: 15-20 grams

Carbohydrates: 5-10 grams (including fiber)

Serving Size: 1 wedge

LECTIN-FRIENDLY SALAD WITH ROASTED BEETS AND VINAIGRETTE

Yield: 2 servings | **Preparation Time:** 10 minutes (plus roasting time for beets, if needed) | **Cooking Time:** 45-60 minutes (for roasting beets, if using raw)

INGREDIENTS

For the Salad:

- 2 cups mixed greens (such as romaine, arugula, spinach)
- 2-3 roasted beets, peeled and sliced (or use pre-cooked beets)
- 1/2 cup chopped cucumber
- 1/4 cup crumbled walnuts or pecans (optional)

For the Lectin-Friendly Vinaigrette:

- 1/4 cup olive oil
- 2 tablespoons apple cider vinegar
- 1 tablespoon balsamic vinegar (optional)
- 1 teaspoon Dijon mustard
- 1/2 teaspoon honey or another lectin-free sweetener (optional)
- To taste, add iodized sea salt and black pepper.

PREPARATION METHODS

1. Roast the Beets (if using raw beets): Preheat the oven to 400°F (200°C). Wrap whole beets in aluminum foil and roast for 45-60 minutes, or until tender when pierced with a fork. Let cool, then peel and slice.
2. Prepare the Salad: In a large bowl, combine mixed greens, sliced beets, chopped cucumber, and walnuts or pecans (optional).
3. Make the Lectin-Friendly Vinaigrette: In a small jar or bowl, whisk together olive oil, apple cider vinegar, balsamic vinegar (optional), Dijon mustard, honey or sweetener (optional), sea salt, and black pepper.
4. Assemble the Salad: Drizzle the vinaigrette over the salad and toss to coat.

TIPS

- For added flavor, marinate the sliced beets in a little balsamic vinegar and olive oil before assembling the salad.

- Experiment with other lectin-free chopped vegetables in the salad, such as shredded carrots, chopped bell peppers (if tolerated), or crumbled cauliflower.

- Lectin-Free Tip: This recipe avoids goat cheese and uses a lectin-friendly vinaigrette with apple cider vinegar instead of ingredients like dairy or tomatoes. You can omit the honey or sweetener if desired for a stricter lectin-free approach.

NUTRITIONAL INFORMATION

Calories: 350-400

Protein: 5-10 grams

Fat: 20-25 grams

Carbohydrates: 20-25 grams (including fiber)

Serving Size: 1 salad

ALMOND FLOUR PANCAKES WITH MIXED BERRY COMPOTE

Yield: 2-3 servings | **Preparation Time:** 10 minutes | **Cooking Time:** 10-15 minutes

INGREDIENTS

For the Pancakes:

- 1 cup almond flour
- 1/4 cup unsweetened shredded coconut (optional)
- 1/4 teaspoon baking powder
- 1/4 teaspoon baking soda
- Iodized sea salt
- 3 large eggs
- 1/4 cup milk alternative (coconut milk, almond milk)
- 1 tablespoon melted coconut oil
- 1 teaspoon vanilla extract (optional)

For the Mixed Berry Compote (optional):

- 1 cup mixed berries (strawberries, blueberries, raspberries)
- 1-2 tablespoons water
- 1 tablespoon lemon juice (optional)
- Pinch of allulose or another lectin-free sweetener (optional)

PREPARATION METHODS

1. Prepare the Pancakes: In a bowl, whisk together almond flour, shredded coconut (optional), baking powder, baking soda, and sea salt.
2. In a separate bowl, whisk together eggs, milk alternative, melted coconut oil, and vanilla extract (optional).
3. Combine the wet and dry ingredients, mixing until just combined. Don't overmix.
4. Heat a lightly greased skillet over medium heat. Pour 1/4 cup batter per pancake.
5. Cook for approximately two to three minutes on each side, or until well cooked and golden brown.
6. When bubbles start to form on the surface, flip.
7. For the Mixed Berry Compote (optional): In a small saucepan, combine berries, water, lemon juice (optional), and sweetener (optional). Heat over medium heat until the berries soften and release their juices, about 5 minutes. Mash slightly with a fork if desired.

TIPS

- For thicker pancakes, use slightly less milk alternative.
- Add a pinch of cinnamon or nutmeg to the batter for extra flavor.
- Top the pancakes with your favorite lectin-free toppings like sliced banana, additional berries, or chopped nuts (almonds, walnuts).
- Lectin-Free Tip: This recipe is naturally lectin-free by avoiding wheat flour and dairy. Substitute regular milk with a lectin-free milk alternative.

NUTRITIONAL INFORMATION

Calories: 300-350

Protein: 20-25 grams

Fat: 20-25 grams

Carbohydrates: 10-15 grams (including fiber)

Serving Size: 2-3 pancakes

CREAMY AVOCADO PASTA WITH SHIRATAKI NOODLES

Yield: 1-2 servings | **Preparation Time:** 5 minutes | **Cooking Time:** No cooking required
(unless pre-cooking shirataki noodles)

INGREDIENTS

- 1 package shirataki noodles (rinsed and drained)
- 1 ripe avocado
- 1/4 cup chopped fresh cilantro
- 1/4 cup chopped fresh parsley
- 1 tablespoon olive oil
- 2 tablespoons lemon juice
- 1 tablespoon water (or more to adjust consistency)
- To taste, add black pepper and iodized sea salt.

PREPARATION METHODS

1. Prepare the Avocado Sauce: In a blender or food processor, combine avocado, cilantro, parsley, olive oil, lemon juice, water, sea salt, and black pepper. Blend until smooth and creamy.
2. Cook the Shirataki Noodles: If desired, follow package instructions to pre-cook the shirataki noodles in boiling water for a few minutes. Drain well.
3. Assemble the Dish: In a large bowl, toss the shirataki noodles with the avocado sauce.
4. If additional water is required to get the right consistency, add it.

- For a richer flavor, add a tablespoon of nutritional yeast to the avocado sauce.
- Experiment with other lectin-free herbs in the sauce, such as chopped chives, basil, or oregano.
- Top the dish with chopped nuts (almonds, walnuts) for added texture and healthy fats.
- Lectin-Free Tip: Shirataki noodles are made from konjac root, a lectin-free ingredient. This recipe avoids dairy by using avocado for creaminess.

NUTRITIONAL INFORMATION

Calories: 200-250

Protein: 5-10 grams

Fat: 15-20 grams

Carbohydrates: 5-10 grams (including fiber)

Serving Size: 1 serving

RAINBOW VEGGIE SKEWERS WITH AVOCADO CHIMICHURRI

Yield: 2-3 servings | **Preparation Time:** 15 minutes | **Cooking Time:** 10-15 minutes (for roasting vegetables, grilling time may vary)

INGREDIENTS

For the Rainbow Veggie Skewers:

- 1 zucchini, cut into chunks
- 1 yellow squash, cut into chunks
- 1 red onion, cut into wedges (optional)
- 1 cup mushrooms, sliced (optional)
- 1 cup broccoli florets
- 1 tablespoon olive oil
- To taste, add black pepper and iodized sea salt.

For the Avocado Chimichurri:

- 1 ripe avocado
- 1/4 cup chopped fresh parsley
- 2 tablespoons chopped fresh cilantro
- 1 tablespoon olive oil
- 2 tablespoons lemon juice
- 1 clove garlic, minced
- To taste, add black pepper and iodized sea salt.

PREPARATION METHODS

1. Prepare the Vegetables: Preheat the oven to 400°F (200°C) if using cherry tomatoes (not recommended for lectin-free). Toss zucchini, yellow squash, red onion (optional), mushrooms (optional), and broccoli florets with olive oil, sea salt, and pepper.

2. Roast the Vegetables (optional): If using cherry tomatoes, spread them on a baking sheet and roast for 10-15 minutes, until slightly softened. Alternatively, precook broccoli florets in boiling water for a few minutes if desired.

3. Assemble the Skewers: Thread the prepared vegetables onto skewers, alternating colors for a rainbow effect.

4. Make the Avocado Chimichurri: In a blender or food processor, combine avocado, parsley, cilantro, olive oil, lemon juice, garlic, sea salt, and pepper. Blend until slightly chunky.

5. Cook the Skewers: Heat a grill pan or grill over medium heat. Grill the skewers for 3-5 minutes per side, or until tender-crisp.

6. Serve the skewers with the avocado chimichurri for dipping.

- Marinate the vegetables in your favorite lectin-free marinade for extra flavor before grilling.

- Feel free to add other lectin-free vegetables to the skewers, such as asparagus spears or eggplant slices.

- For a smoky flavor, add a few drops of liquid smoke to the avocado chimichurri.

NUTRITIONAL INFORMATION

Calories: 300-350

Protein: 5-10 grams

Fat: 20-25 grams

Carbohydrates: 15-20 grams (including fiber)

Serving Size: 1 serving with skewers and chimichurri

SWEET POTATO AND SAUSAGE FRITTATA WITH KALE AND ONIONS

Yield: 4-6 servings | **Preparation Time:** 15 minutes | **Cooking Time:** 30-35 minutes

INGREDIENTS

- 1 medium sweet potato, peeled and diced
- 1 tablespoon olive oil
- 1/2 onion, chopped
- 4 ounces ground turkey or chicken sausage (casings removed)
- 4 cups chopped kale, stems removed
- 8 large eggs, beaten
- 1/4 cup chopped fresh parsley
- To taste, add black pepper and iodized sea salt.

PREPARATION METHODS

1. Preheat the oven to 375°F (190°C). Grease a pie plate or an oven-safe 10-inch skillet.
2. Cook the Sweet Potato: In a large skillet, heat olive oil over medium heat. Add the diced sweet potato and cook for 5-7 minutes, or until slightly softened. Set aside.
3. Sauté the Onion and Sausage: In the same skillet, add the chopped onion and cook for 2-3 minutes, until softened. Add the ground turkey or chicken sausage and cook until browned, breaking it up with a spoon as it cooks.
4. Incorporate Kale: Stir in the chopped kale and cook for another minute, or until wilted.
5. Assemble the Frittata: In a large bowl, whisk together the beaten eggs, chopped parsley, sea salt, and black pepper. Add the cooked sweet potato mixture and sausage-kale mixture to the egg mixture.

6. Bake the Frittata: Pour the mixture into the greased skillet or pie dish. Bake for 25-30 minutes, or until the eggs are set and the center is no longer runny.

7. Let cool slightly before slicing and serving.

TIPS

- For a vegetarian option, omit the sausage and add another cup of chopped vegetables, such as mushrooms or zucchini.
- Feel free to use other herbs in place of parsley, such as chopped chives or thyme.
- Top the frittata with your favorite lectin-free toppings like sliced avocado or additional chopped fresh herbs.
- Lectin-Free Tip: This recipe avoids nightshade vegetables (tomatoes) and dairy products. Use ground turkey or chicken sausage for a lectin-free protein source.

NUTRITIONAL INFORMATION

Calories: 350-400

Protein: 25-30 grams

Fat: 15-20 grams

Carbohydrates: 20-25 grams (including fiber)

Serving Size: 1 wedge

LECTIN-FRIENDLY GREEN SMOOTHIE BOWL WITH BERRIES

Yield: 1 serving | **Preparation Time:** 5 minutes | **Cooking Time:** No cooking required

INGREDIENTS

- One cup of unsweetened coconut or almond milk
- One cup of frozen berry mixture (raspberries, blueberries, and strawberries)
- 1 handful chopped spinach
- 1/2 banana (optional, for sweetness)
- Iodized sea salt (optional)

Optional Toppings (avoid chia seeds for strict lectin-free):

- Coconut flakes
- Sliced almonds
- Additional berries

PREPARATION METHODS

1. In a blender, combine almond milk or coconut milk, frozen berries, spinach, and banana (optional). Blend until smooth and creamy.
2. Pour the smoothie into a bowl.
3. Top with your favorite lectin-free toppings: coconut flakes, sliced almonds, or additional berries.

- Experiment with other lectin-free fruits and vegetables in the smoothie, such as chopped mango or frozen cauliflower.
- Add a scoop of collagen peptides (optional, if tolerated) for an extra protein boost.
- Adjust the thickness of the smoothie by adding more or less almond milk or coconut milk.
- Lectin-Free Tip: This recipe omits chia seeds, which are high in lectins. Enjoy the refreshing combination of berries, spinach, and almond milk or coconut milk.

NUTRITIONAL INFORMATION

Calories: 200-250

Protein: 5-10 grams

Fat: 5-10 grams

Carbohydrates: 25-30 grams (including fiber)

Serving Size: 1 bowl

FRITTATA WITH SAUTEED MUSHROOMS AND SPINACH

Yield: 4-6 servings | **Preparation Time:** 10 minutes | **Cooking Time:** 25-30 minutes

INGREDIENTS

- 8 large eggs
- 1/4 cup chopped fresh parsley
- To taste, add iodized sea salt and black pepper.
- 1 tablespoon olive oil
- 8 ounces sliced mushrooms (cremini, portobello, or your choice)
- 4 cups chopped fresh spinach

PREPARATION METHODS

1. Preheat the oven to 375°F (190°C). Coat a 10-inch oven-safe skillet or pie plate with grease.
2. Whisk the Eggs: In a large bowl, whisk together eggs, parsley, sea salt, and black pepper.
3. Sauté the Mushrooms: Heat olive oil in the skillet over medium heat. Add the sliced mushrooms and cook for 5-7 minutes, or until softened and golden brown.
4. Incorporate Spinach: Stir in the chopped spinach and cook for another minute, or until wilted.
5. Assemble and Bake the Frittata: Pour the egg mixture over the cooked vegetables in the skillet. Bake for 20-25 minutes, or until the eggs are set and the center is no longer runny.
6. Let cool slightly before slicing and serving.

- For a vegetarian option, add crumbled cooked tempeh or chopped roasted vegetables to the egg mixture.
- Feel free to use other herbs in place of parsley, such as chopped chives or thyme.
- Top the frittata with your favorite lectin-free toppings like sliced avocado or additional chopped fresh herbs.
- Lectin-Free Tip: This recipe avoids tomatoes (typically used in omelets) and dairy products. It offers a lectin-friendly alternative with a focus on mushrooms and spinach.

NUTRITIONAL INFORMATION

Calories: 250-300

Protein: 20-25 grams

Fat: 15-20 grams

Carbohydrates: 5-10 grams (including fiber)

Serving Size: 1 wedge

ALMOND FLOUR MUFFINS WITH BERRIES AND COCONUT MILK

Yield: 6-8 muffins | **Preparation Time:** 15 minutes | **Cooking Time:** 18-20 minutes

INGREDIENTS

For the Muffins:

- 1 1/2 cups almond flour
- 1/4 cup unsweetened shredded coconut (optional)
- 1/2 teaspoon baking powder
- 1/4 teaspoon baking soda
- Iodized sea salt
- 3 large eggs
- 1/3 cup melted coconut oil
- 1/3 cup maple syrup or another lectin-free sweetener (like allulose)
- 1/2 cup unsweetened coconut milk

PREPARATION METHODS

1. Preheat the oven to 350°F (175°C). Line a muffin tin with paper liners.
2. Whisk Dry Ingredients: In a medium bowl, whisk together almond flour, shredded coconut (optional), baking powder, baking soda, and sea salt.
3. Whisk Wet Ingredients: In a separate bowl, whisk together eggs, melted coconut oil, maple syrup (or alternative sweetener), and coconut milk.
4. Combine Wet and Dry Ingredients: Add the wet ingredients to the dry ingredients and mix until just combined. Don't overmix.
5. Fold in Berries: Gently fold in the mixed berries.
6. Fill the Muffin Tin: Divide batter evenly among the prepared muffin cups.

7. A toothpick inserted in the center should come out clean after baking for approximately eighteen to twenty minutes.

8. Let cool slightly before serving.

TIPS

- For a moister muffin, add a mashed banana to the batter.
- Substitute a portion of the almond flour with coconut flour (use 1/3 cup coconut flour and 1 cup almond flour) for a different texture.
- Top the muffins with additional berries or chopped nuts (almonds, walnuts) before baking.
- Lectin-Free Tip:
  - This recipe is naturally lectin-free by avoiding wheat flour and dairy. Coconut milk and berries are lectin-friendly options.
  - This recipe avoids nightshade vegetables (tomatoes) and dairy products. Use ground turkey or chicken sausage for a lectin-free protein source.

NUTRITIONAL INFORMATION

Calories: 350-400

Protein: 10-15 grams

Fat: 20-25 grams

Carbohydrates: 20-25 grams (includ ing fiber)

Serving Size: 1 muffin

PAN-SEARED SCALLOPS WITH CREAMY AVOCADO SAUCE

Yield: 2-3 servings | **Preparation Time:** 10 minutes | **Cooking Time:** 5-7 minutes

INGREDIENTS

For the Scallops:

- 1 pound sea scallops (dry sea scallops are recommended)
- 1 tablespoon olive oil
- To taste, add black pepper and iodized sea salt.

For the Creamy Avocado Sauce:

- 1 ripe avocado
- 1/4 cup chopped fresh cilantro
- 1/4 cup chopped fresh parsley
- 2 tablespoons lemon juice
- 1 tablespoon olive oil
- To taste, add black pepper and iodized sea salt.

PREPARATION METHODS

1. Prepare the Scallops by using paper towels to pat them dry.
2. Season them lightly with sea salt and black pepper.
3. Heat the Oil: Heat olive oil in a large skillet over medium-high heat.
4. Sear the Scallops: Sear the scallops for 2-3 minutes per side, or until golden brown and cooked through. They might turn rubbery if you overcook them, so handle with caution.
5. Make the Avocado Sauce: While the scallops are cooking, in a blender or food processor, combine avocado, chopped cilantro, chopped parsley, lemon juice, olive oil, sea salt, and pepper. Blend until smooth and creamy.

6. Serve: Plate the seared scallops and top them with the creamy avocado sauce.

TIPS

- For a richer sauce, add a tablespoon of nutritional yeast to the avocado mixture.
- If the avocado sauce is too thick, add a tablespoon of water or coconut milk to thin it out.
- Serve the scallops and sauce over a bed of roasted vegetables for a more complete meal.
- Lectin-Free Tip: This recipe avoids dairy products by using avocado for creaminess. Scallops are naturally lectin-free.

NUTRITIONAL INFORMATION

Calories: 400-450 (estimates will vary depending on specific ingredients used)

Protein: 30-35 grams

Fat: 25-30 grams

Carbohydrates: 5-10 grams (including fiber)

Serving Size: 1 serving (scallops with sauce)

SUNSHINE CITRUS SHRIMP SKEWERS WITH COCONUT LIME GLAZE

Yield: 2-3 servings | **Preparation Time:** 15 minutes (plus marinating time) | **Cooking Time:** 5-7 minutes

INGREDIENTS

For the Skewers:

- 1 pound large raw shrimp, peeled and deveined (tails on or off, your preference)
- 1 tablespoon olive oil
- 1/2 lemon, juiced (about 2 tablespoons)
- 1/4 cup chopped fresh parsley
- 1 clove garlic, minced
- To taste, add black pepper and iodized sea salt.
- 1 zucchini, cut into chunks (optional)
- 1 yellow squash, cut into chunks (optional)

For the Coconut Lime Glaze:

- 1/4 cup unsweetened coconut milk
- 1 tablespoon lime juice
- 1 tablespoon honey or another lectin-free sweetener (like allulose)
- 1 tablespoon chopped fresh cilantro

PREPARATION METHODS

1. Marinate the Shrimp: In a large bowl, combine olive oil, lemon juice, parsley, garlic, sea salt, and black pepper. Add the shrimp and toss to coat. Let it marinate for a minimum of half an hour or for as long as two hours in the fridge.
2. Prepare the Glaze (optional): In a small saucepan, whisk together coconut milk, lime juice, sweetener, and cilantro. Heat over low heat until simmering, then remove from heat.
3. Prepare the Skewers (optional): To avoid burning, soak wooden skewers in water for at least half an hour.

4. Thread the shrimp on skewers, alternating with zucchini and yellow squash chunks (optional).

5. Cook the Shrimp: Preheat the oven to broil or grill over medium-high heat. Broil or grill the skewers for 2-3 minutes per side, or until the shrimp are pink and cooked through.

6. Glaze the Shrimp (optional): Brush the cooked shrimp with the coconut lime glaze (optional) during the last minute of cooking.

TIPS

- For a smoky flavor, add a teaspoon of smoked paprika to the marinade.

- You can use other citrus fruits in the marinade, such as orange juice or grapefruit juice.

- If not using skewers, simply cook the shrimp in a skillet over medium heat until cooked through.

- Lectin-Free Tip: This recipe avoids all lectin-heavy ingredients. Shrimp, citrus fruits, coconut milk, and herbs are all lectin-free friendly. The glaze is optional, but if using it, choose a lectin-free sweetener like allulose or monk fruit sweetener.

NUTRITIONAL INFORMATION

Calories: 300-350

Protein: 30-35 grams

Fat: 10-15 grams

Carbohydrates: 5-10 grams (including fiber)

Serving Size: 1 serving (shrimp with optional glaze)

ZESTY BERRIES AND AVOCADO SALAD WITH TOASTED PECANS

Yield: 2 servings | **Preparation Time:** 10 minutes | **Cooking Time:** Toasting pecans takes 5-7 minutes (optional)

INGREDIENTS

For the Salad:

- 2 cups mixed berries (strawberries, blueberries, raspberries)
- 1 ripe avocado, diced
- 1/2 cup chopped romaine lettuce or baby spinach
- 1/4 cup crumbled goat cheese (optional, omit for stricter lectin-free)
- 1/4 cup chopped pecans, toasted
- To taste, add black pepper and iodized sea salt.

For the Dressing (optional):

- 2 tablespoons olive oil
- 1 tablespoon lemon juice
- 1 tablespoon balsamic vinegar (optional, omit for stricter lectin-free)
- 1/2 teaspoon Dijon mustard
- To taste, add black pepper and iodized sea salt.

PREPARATION METHODS

1. Prepare the Salad: In a large bowl, combine mixed berries, diced avocado, romaine lettuce or spinach, goat cheese (optional), and toasted pecans.
2. Make the Dressing (optional): In a small jar or bowl, whisk together olive oil, lemon juice, balsamic vinegar (optional), Dijon mustard, sea salt, and pepper.
3. Dress the Salad (optional): Drizzle the dressing over the salad before serving, or serve dressing on the side for individual control.

- For a sweeter salad, add a drizzle of honey or another lectin-free sweetener before serving.
- Substitute the pecans with another lectin-free nut or seed, such as sliced almonds or hemp seeds (avoid for stricter lectin-free).
- For a more substantial salad, add grilled chicken or fish on top.
- Lectin-Free Tip: Berries, avocado, lettuce/spinach, and olive oil are all lectin-free friendly. Goat cheese is optional, and some people tolerate goat and sheep dairy on a lectin-free diet. If following a stricter lectin-free approach, omit the goat cheese and balsamic vinegar.

NUTRITIONAL INFORMATION

Calories: 400-450 (estimates will vary depending on specific ingredients used)

Protein: 10-15 grams

Fat: 25-30 grams

Carbohydrates: 20-25 grams (including fiber)

Serving Size: 1 salad

HERB-CRUSTED SALMON WITH ROASTED ASPARAGUS AND LEMON BUTTER

Yield: 2 servings | **Preparation Time:** 10 minutes | **Cooking Time:** 15-20 minutes

INGREDIENTS

For the Salmon:

- 2 salmon filets (about 6 ounces each)
- 2 tablespoons olive oil
- 1/4 cup chopped fresh herbs (such as parsley, dill, and thyme)
- 1 tablespoon almond flour or coconut flour
- To taste, add black pepper and iodized sea salt.

For the Roasted Asparagus:

- 1 pound asparagus spears, trimmed
- 1 tablespoon olive oil
- To taste, add black pepper and iodized sea salt.
- For the Lemon Butter (optional):
- 2 tablespoons unsalted butter (or ghee)
- 1 tablespoon lemon juice
- 1/4 teaspoon chopped fresh parsley

PREPARATION METHODS

1. Preheat the oven to 400°F (200°C).
2. Prepare the Salmon: In a shallow dish, combine olive oil, chopped herbs, almond flour or coconut flour, sea salt, and pepper. Pat the salmon filets dry and coat them in the herb mixture.
3. Roast the Asparagus: Toss the asparagus spears with olive oil, sea salt, and pepper. Arrange them in a solitary layer on an oven tray.
4. Bake the Salmon and Asparagus: Place the salmon filets on a separate baking sheet. Roast the salmon and asparagus for 15-20 minutes, or until the salmon is cooked through and the asparagus is tender-crisp.
5. Make the Lemon Butter (optional): While the salmon and asparagus are cooking, in a small saucepan over low heat, melt the butter (or ghee). Take off the heat and mix in the chopped parsley and lemon juice.
6. Serve: Plate the roasted asparagus and top with the herb-crusted salmon. Drizzle with lemon butter (optional) before serving.

- Use a variety of your favorite fresh herbs for the salmon crust.
- If you don't have almond flour or coconut flour, you can use panko breadcrumbs for the crust, but this is not lectin-free.
- Serve the salmon and asparagus with a side of roasted sweet potato wedges or cauliflower rice for a more complete meal.
- Lectin-Free Tip: Salmon, asparagus, olive oil, lemon juice, and herbs are all lectin-free friendly. Lemon butter is optional, and butter is generally tolerated on a lectin-free diet. If avoiding dairy entirely, substitute ghee or coconut oil for butter.

NUTRITIONAL INFORMATION

Calories: 500-550

Protein: 40-45 grams

Fat: 30-35 grams

Carbohydrates: 15-20 grams (including fiber)

Serving Size: 1 serving (salmon with asparagus and optional lemon butter)

COCONUT CURRY CAULIFLOWER RICE BOWLS WITH CILANTRO LIME SHRIMP

Yield: 2-3 servings | **Preparation Time:** 15 minutes | **Cooking Time:** 15-20 minutes

INGREDIENTS

- For the Coconut Curry:
- 1 tablespoon olive oil
- 1 tablespoon curry powder
- 1/2 teaspoon ground ginger
- 1/4 teaspoon turmeric
- 1 can (13.5 oz) coconut milk
- 1 cup vegetable broth
- To taste, add black pepper and iodized sea salt.
- 1 tablespoon chopped fresh cilantro (optional)

For the Cauliflower Rice:

- 1 head cauliflower, riced (using a food processor or box grater)
- 1 tablespoon olive oil
- To taste, add black pepper and iodized sea salt.

For the Cilantro Lime Shrimp:

- 1 pound raw shrimp, peeled and deveined (tails on or off)
- 1 tablespoon olive oil
- 1/2 lime, juiced (about 2 tablespoons)
- 1/4 cup chopped fresh cilantro
- 1 clove garlic, minced
- To taste, add black pepper and iodized sea salt.

PREPARATION METHODS

1. Make the Coconut Curry: In a medium saucepan, heat olive oil over medium heat. Add curry powder, ginger, and turmeric and cook for 30 seconds, stirring constantly, to release the flavors.
2. Whisk in Coconut Milk and Broth: Stir in coconut milk and vegetable broth.
3. Cook for five minutes, or until moderately thickened, after bringing to a simmer.
4. Use black pepper and sea salt for seasoning.

5. Add chopped cilantro (optional) for extra flavor.

6. Cook the Cauliflower Rice: In a large skillet, heat olive oil over medium heat. Add the riced cauliflower and cook for 5-7 minutes, or until tender-crisp, stirring occasionally.

7. Use black pepper and sea salt for seasoning.

8. Cook the Cilantro Lime Shrimp: While the cauliflower rice cooks, in a separate skillet, heat olive oil over medium-high heat.

9. Cook the shrimp for two to three minutes on each side, or until they are cooked through and pink.

10. Stir in lime juice, chopped cilantro, and minced garlic during the last minute of cooking. Season with sea salt and black pepper.

11. Assemble the Bowls: Divide the cauliflower rice between bowls. Top with the coconut curry, cilantro lime shrimp, and additional fresh cilantro (optional).

TIPS

- For a vegetarian option, omit the shrimp and add roasted vegetables like broccoli or bell peppers (avoid red peppers for strict lectin-free).
- You can adjust the curry powder to your desired level of spice.
- Serve the bowls with a squeeze of lime juice for extra flavor.
- Lectin-Free Tip: This recipe avoids all lectin-heavy ingredients. Coconut milk, vegetables, herbs, and shrimp are all lectin-free friendly.

NUTRITIONAL INFORMATION

Calories: 450-500

Protein: 40-45 grams

Fat: 20-25 grams

Carbohydrates: 25-30 grams (including fiber)

Serving Size: 1 bowl

LECTIN-FRIENDLY KOREAN BEEF BOWLS WITH SESAME GINGER VINAIGRETTE AND LETTUCE WRAPS

Yield: 2-3 servings | **Preparation Time:** 15 minutes | **Cooking Time:** 10-12 minutes

INGREDIENTS

For the Lectin-Friendly Korean Beef:

- 1 pound ground beef (or ground turkey)
- 1 tablespoon coconut aminos
- 1 tablespoon sesame oil
- 1 tablespoon soy sauce (use tamari for a gluten-free option) - omit for stricter lectin-free
- 1/2 teaspoon ground ginger
- 1/4 teaspoon garlic powder
- To taste, add black pepper and iodized sea salt.

For the Sesame Ginger Vinaigrette:

- 2 tablespoons olive oil
- 1 tablespoon rice vinegar (or apple cider vinegar)
- 1 tablespoon toasted sesame oil
- 1 tablespoon soy sauce (use tamari for a gluten-free option) - omit for stricter lectin-free
- 1/2 teaspoon grated ginger
- 1 clove garlic, minced
- To taste, add black pepper and iodized sea salt.

For the Lettuce Wraps:

- One head of washed and sorted romaine lettuce

PREPARATION METHODS

1. Make the Lectin-Friendly Korean Beef: In a large bowl, combine ground beef (or turkey), coconut aminos, sesame oil, soy sauce (use tamari for a gluten-free option, omit for stricter lectin-free), ginger powder, garlic powder, sea salt, and pepper. Mix well.

2. Cook the Beef: Turn up the heat to moderate in a big skillet. Add the beef mixture and cook for 5-7 minutes, or until browned and cooked through, breaking it up with a spoon as it cooks. Drain any excess grease.

3. Make the Sesame Ginger Vinaigrette (optional): In a small jar or bowl, whisk together olive oil, rice vinegar (or apple cider vinegar), toasted sesame oil, soy sauce (use tamari for

a gluten-free option, omit for stricter lectin-free), grated ginger, minced garlic, sea salt, and pepper.

4. Assemble the Bowls and Wraps: Divide the cooked Korean beef between bowls. Top with desired toppings like chopped green onions, shredded carrots, or kimchi (avoid if following a stricter lectin-free approach). Drizzle with sesame ginger vinaigrette (optional). Serve with romaine lettuce leaves for wrapping.

TIPS

- For a spicier flavor, add a pinch of red pepper flakes to the Korean beef mixture.
- You can substitute ground chicken or pork for ground beef or turkey.
- Serve the bowls with a side of cauliflower rice for a more complete meal.
- Lectin-Free Tip: This recipe is mostly lectin-friendly. Coconut aminos, sesame oil, ginger, garlic, and lettuce are all lectin-free. Soy sauce (or tamari) is included for an optional flavor but can be omitted for a stricter lectin-free approach. Kimchi often contains red peppers, so avoid it if following stricter lectin-free.

NUTRITIONAL INFORMATION

Calories: 400-450 (without vinaigrette)

Protein: 40-45 grams

Fat: 20-25 grams

Carbohydrates: 10-15 grams (including fiber)

Serving Size: 1 bowl with lettuce wraps

TROPICAL GREEN SMOOTHIE BOWL

Yield: 1 serving | **Preparation Time:** 5 minutes | **Cooking Time:** No cooking required

INGREDIENTS

For the Smoothie Base:

- 2 cups unsweetened almond milk or coconut milk
- 1 handful frozen spinach
- One cup of frozen berry mixture (raspberries, blueberries, and strawberries)
- 1/2 ripe avocado
- 1 tablespoon lime juice
- 1 scoop vanilla protein powder (optional)

For the Toppings (choose lectin-free options):

- Sliced banana or berries
- Shredded coconut
- Chopped nuts or seeds (almonds, walnuts - avoid for stricter lectin-free)
- Hemp seeds (avoid for stricter lectin-free)

PREPARATION METHODS

1. Blend the Smoothie Base: In a high-powered blender, combine almond milk (or coconut milk), spinach, frozen berries, avocado, lime juice, and protein powder (optional). Blend until smooth and creamy.

2. Assemble the Bowl: Pour the smoothie base into a bowl. Top with your favorite lectin-free toppings like sliced banana, berries, shredded coconut, chopped nuts (avoid for stricter lectin-free), or hemp seeds (avoid for stricter lectin-free).

TIPS

- Feel free to adjust the sweetness of the smoothie by adding a little honey or another lectin-free sweetener.
- You can add a scoop of nut butter (avoid cashews for lectin-free) for extra protein and healthy fats.
- For a thicker smoothie bowl, use less liquid or add a frozen banana.

NUTRITIONAL INFORMATION

Calories: 300-350

Protein: 15-20 grams (with protein powder)

Fat: 10-15 grams

Carbohydrates: 25-30 grams (including fiber)

Serving Size: 1 bowl

Chapter 5

Day	Breakfast	Lunch	Dinner	Snack	Category (pg #)
Day 1	Sweet Potato and Sausage Frittata with Kale and Onions (pg. 55)	Spicy Shrimp Stir-Fry with Broccoli and Coconut Aminos (pg. 21) with a side salad	Coconut Curry Chicken with Cauliflower Rice (pg. 33)	Almond Flour Muffins with Berries and Coconut Milk (pg. 61)	4, 1, 2, 4
Day 2	Lectin-Friendly Green Smoothie Bowl with Berries (pg. 57)	Leftover Coconut Curry Chicken with Cauliflower Rice (pg. 33)	Baked Cod with Lemon and Artichokes (pg. 23) with roasted vegetables	Coconut Flour Pancakes with Mixed Berry Compote (pg. 43)	4, 2, 1, 3
Day 3	Mushroom and Spinach Omelet with Roasted Tomatoes (pg. 59)	Marinated Chicken Fajita Salad with Cilantro Lime Dressing (pg. 41)	Thai Green Curry with Shrimp and Broccoli (pg. 25)	Zesty Berries and Avocado Salad with Toasted Pecans (pg. 67)	4, 2, 1, 5
Day 4	Almond Flour Pancakes with Mixed Berry Compote (pg. 49)	Leftover Thai Green Curry with Shrimp and Broccoli (pg. 25)	Seared Chicken with Garlic Green Beans and Mashed Sweet Potatoes (pg. 31)	Tropical Green Smoothie Bowl (pg. 75)	3, 1, 2, 5

Day 5	Frittata with Sauteed Mushrooms and Spinach (pg. 45)	Shrimp Scampi with Shirataki Noodles and Garlic (pg. 27)	One-Pan Chicken Fajitas with Onions (pg. 39) with cauliflower rice	Lectin-Friendly Salad with Roasted Beets and Vinaigrette (pg. 47)	3, 1, 2, 3
Day 6	Pan-Seared Scallops with Creamy Avocado Sauce (pg. 62)	Leftover One-Pan Chicken Fajitas with Onions (pg. 39)	Herb-Crusted Salmon with Roasted Brussels Sprouts and Avocado Salsa (pg. 19)	Creamy Avocado Pasta with Shirataki Noodles (pg. 63)	4, 2, 1, 3
Day 7	Rest Day	Choose your favorite breakfast option from the previous days			
Day 8	Lectin-Friendly Green Smoothie Bowl with Berries (pg. 57)	Spicy Chicken Lettuce Wraps with Sweet Potato Fries (pg. 37)	Coconut Curry Mussels with Sweet Potato Noodles (pg. 29)	Almond Flour Muffins with Berries and Coconut Milk (pg. 61)	4, 2, 1, 4
Day 9	Sweet Potato and Sausage Frittata with Kale and Onions (pg. 55)	Leftover Coconut Curry Mussels with Sweet Potato Noodles (pg. 29)	Turmeric-Roasted Chicken with Parsnips and Carrots (pg. 35)	Zesty Berries and Avocado Salad with Toasted Pecans (pg. 67)	4, 1, 2, 5

Day 10	Mushroom and Spinach Omelet with Roasted Tomatoes (pg. 59)	Herb-Crusted Salmon with Roasted Asparagus and Lemon Butter (pg. 69) with a side salad	Coconut Flour Pancakes with Mixed Berry Compote (pg. 43)	Tropical Green Smoothie Bowl (pg. 75)	4, 5, 3, 5
Day 11	Almond Flour Pancakes with Mixed Berry Compote (pg. 49)	Leftover Turmeric-Roasted Chicken with Parsnips and Carrots (pg. 35)	Baked Cod with Lemon and Artichokes (pg. 23) with roasted vegetables	Lectin-Friendly Salad with Roasted Beets and Vinaigrette (pg. 47)	3, 2, 1, 3
Day 12	Frittata with Sauteed Mushrooms and Spinach (pg. 45)	Sunshine Citrus Shrimp Skewers with Coconut Lime Glaze (pg. 65) with a side salad	Seared Chicken with Garlic Green Beans and Mashed Sweet Potatoes (pg. 31)	Creamy Avocado Pasta with Shirataki Noodles (pg. 63)	3, 5, 2, 3
Day 13	Rest Day	Leftover Sunshine Citrus Shrimp Skewers with Coconut Lime Glaze (pg. 65)	Thai Green Curry with Shrimp and Broccoli (pg. 25)	Tropical Green Smoothie Bowl (pg. 75)	
Day 14	Pan-Seared Scallops with Creamy Avocado Sauce (pg. 62)	Leftover Thai Green Curry with Shrimp and Broccoli (pg. 25)	Spicy Chicken Lettuce Wraps with Sweet Potato Fries (pg. 37)	Zesty Berries and Avocado Salad with Toasted Pecans (pg. 67)	4, 1, 2, 5

Tips:

- Feel free to swap lunches and dinners throughout the week to create variety.
- Leftovers are a great way to save time and avoid food waste.
- Adjust portion sizes based on your individual needs.
- Experiment with different lectin-free ingredients and flavors to create your own delicious meals.
- This is just a sample plan; feel free to get creative and incorporate your favorite lectin-free recipes.

Chapter 6

Sticking to a lectin-free diet while dining out or attending social gatherings can feel challenging. Fear not, fellow lectin-free friends! This guide equips you with strategies and sample options to navigate various restaurant settings:

General Tips:

Plan Ahead: Research menus online beforehand. Identify lectin-free friendly options or dishes that can be easily modified.

Communicate Clearly: Inform your server about your dietary restrictions and ask questions about ingredients. Don't hesitate to ask for substitutions.

Be Prepared: Pack snacks like nuts (avoid cashews for stricter lectin-free), sliced vegetables, or fruits (berries are best) in case limited options are available.

Restaurant Types:

Fast Food:

Focus on: Salads with grilled chicken or fish (avoid dressings with added sugar or thickeners), grilled burgers without buns (wrap in lettuce), sugar-free iced tea or water.

Avoid: Breaded items, french fries, sugary drinks, processed deli meats.

Casual Dining:

Appetizers: Opt for grilled shrimp, steamed vegetables with olive oil and herbs, guacamole with chopped vegetables.

Main Courses: Grilled salmon or chicken with steamed vegetables, bunless burgers with lettuce wraps, steak with a side salad (avoid candied toppings).

Sides: Skip the french fries, mashed potatoes, and onion rings. Choose steamed vegetables, side salads with simple vinaigrette, or baked sweet potato (avoid candied toppings).

Ethnic Cuisine:

Italian: Grilled fish or chicken with steamed vegetables, side salad with olive oil and vinegar dressing, minestrone soup (avoid creamy soups).

Mexican: Grilled fish tacos with corn tortillas (avoid flour tortillas), fajita bowls with grilled meat, chicken, or shrimp, side salad with salsa or guacamole.

Asian: Steamed or grilled fish or chicken with stir-fried vegetables (hold the sugary sauces), sushi with various fish options (avoid teriyaki sauce), bunless lettuce wraps with grilled meat or vegetables.

Indian: Tandoori chicken or fish, vegetable curries made with coconut milk (avoid chickpea-based curries), lentil soup (dal) if tolerated.

Social Gatherings:

Offer to Bring a Dish: This way, you have control over ingredients and can ensure a lectin-free option. Consider a crowd-pleasing dish like a lectin-free salad, vegetable platter with guacamole, or a frittata.

Communicate with the Host: Let them know about your dietary restrictions and ask if there might be lectin-free options available.

Focus on Enjoying the Company: Don't stress about food. Focus on socializing and having a good time. You can always eat before or after the event.

Bonus Tip: Download a lectin-free reference app or chart to have a handy guide of lectin-containing foods at your fingertips.

CONCLUSION

ongratulations on taking charge of your health and exploring the world of lectin-free eating! This journey may seem daunting at first, but with the knowledge you've gained from this book, you're well-equipped to navigate the exciting world of lectin-free cuisine.

Remember, this is not just a diet; it's a chance to explore new flavors, rediscover the power of whole foods, and experience a newfound vibrancy in your health. Embrace the lectin-free lifestyle as an opportunity for culinary exploration, not restriction.

This book has served as your guide, but the real adventure starts now. Experiment with new recipes, discover hidden gems at restaurants, and share the lectin-free love with friends and family.

As you set off on this adventure, keep in mind these important advice:

Focus on Abundance: There's a whole world of delicious and nutritious lectin-free foods waiting to be discovered.

Listen to Your Body: Pay attention to how you feel after consuming certain foods and adjust accordingly.

Celebrate Every Milestone: Every healthy choice is a victory!

We hope this book has empowered you to make informed decisions about your lectin-free journey. As you continue to explore, remember, we're all in this together. There's a supportive lectin-free community waiting to welcome you with open arms and share their experiences.

So, grab your favorite lectin-free ingredients, fire up the kitchen, and get ready to experience the transformative power of lectin-free living!

Happy eating, and happy healing!